The Healthiest Shopping List

2ⁿᵈ Edition

43 Healthiest Supermarket Finds Revealed!

by Olivia Rogers

Copyright © 2017 By Olivia Rogers
All rights reserved. No part of this book may be reproduced in any form without permission in writing from the author. No part of this publication may be reproduced or transmitted in any form or by any means, mechanic, electronic, photocopying, recording, by any storage or retrieval system, or transmitted by email without the permission in writing from the author and publisher.
For information regarding permissions write to author at Olivia@TheMenuAtHome.com
Reviewers may quote brief passages in review.

Please note that credit for the images used in this book go to the respective owners. You can view this at:
TheMenuAtHome.com/image-list

Olivia Rogers
TheMenuAtHome.com

Table of Contents

INTRODUCTION — 4

CHAPTER 1: HEALTHY VEGGIES AND FRUITS — 6

CHAPTER 2: HEALTHY PROTEINS — 15

CHAPTER 3: HEALTHY DRINKS — 20

CHAPTER 4: HEALTHY WHOLE GRAINS — 23

CHAPTER 5: HEALTHY DAIRY — 25

FINAL WORDS — 27

DISCLAIMER — 29

Introduction

The generally held belief that our supermarkets are stuffed with unhealthy, canned foods imported from God-knows-where is absolutely misleading. This e-book proves, without an iota of doubt that there are plenty of foods and other related edible products in our supermarkets that are indeed healthy and highly recommendable for everyone's consumption.

Highlighted in this e-book are some great, rare finds that include foods, fruits, vegetables and drinks of different kinds. The criteria for selecting the ones included in this e-book are based on five essential factors:

- They contain life-enriching nutrients and vitamins that are required in day-to-day metabolic activities.

- They contain little calories and hence cannot cause fattening in human bodies.

- They are naturally or organically made: but when they required some additives, in case of some desserts, very limited quantities of food additives were used.

- They are available in supermarkets across the globe; you can find these foods, drinks, vegetables and fruits near you.

- They are affordable and a little quantity of them can produce significant, healthy results in your body.

So, next time you walk into a supermarket, have it in your mind that the place actually holds some great finds you can buy to improve your health, maintain your weight and live a long life.

You don't have to bother yourself about drawing up the appropriate healthy shopping list anymore; we have done the hard job for you by researching at supermarkets which foods, drinks, proteins, fruits and vegetables will possibly improve your health and that of your loved ones. It is an effort that took us some years before we finally settled on these 43 recipes that will surely have some positive impacts on your health.

Enjoy this rare healthy shopping list!

Chapter 1: Healthy Veggies and Fruits

Vegetables and fruits are known to be sources of some minerals and vitamins (most especially, Vitamins K and C) that human bodies need to function properly. Examples of minerals that are found in vegetables and fruits include folic acid, potassium, iron and magnesium.

We have been quite pragmatic in choosing those vegetables and fruits that are capable of replenishing the shortage of minerals and vitamins in your body and give you nothing but sound health.

Relax but be excited about this list of health-improving veggies and fruits you can lay your hand on at any supermarket near you.

The first eight listings are healthy fruits, while the last twelve listings are healthy veggies:

Grapes

Grapes contain high quantity of antioxidants and they are useful for reducing cholesterol. You can get them for cheap prices and they are available all year round! It doesn't matter if they are green or purple ones. You can have them alongside salad and other fruits.

Apples

Do you know why people say eating an apple a day will keep doctors away? This superfood is rich in Vitamin C and antioxidants that can actively fight cancer for you! The red apples seem to be more popular than the green ones, but there is no research finding to prove that red apples are indeed more nutritious than the green ones.

Bananas

Bananas are low-calorie "snacks", and they are rich in fiber and potassium. Fibers are essential facilitators of metabolism in human bodies. And bananas also contain some amount of water which, when eaten, becomes part of the water in human body. Potassium is an element that normally helps lower the risks of blood pressure, stroke and heart disease. In other words, if you consume banana on a regular basis, you are preparing your body to be ready against diseases like cardiac arrest and stroke.

Kiwi

Kiwis are indeed an example of berries and they contain fiber and Vitamin C. Vitamin C is generally helpful in maintaining the cell growth and forms a useful protein in skin, ligament, blood vessels and tendons. The fiber part of kiwi fruits is essential for speeding up the metabolism in human body. You can have your kiwi before or after each meal, depending on your preferences.

Cantaloupe

Cantaloupe is very rich in Vitamin C and they are cheap to obtain. You can be rest assured that the antioxidants a cantaloupe contains can help you maintain a healthy body by slowing your aging process as well as protecting you against any heart disease. If you like, you can mix your cantaloupe with other fruits and vegetables in a bowl of salad.

Watermelons

Watermelons are another example of superfoods, and they contain in large quantities Vitamin C and antioxidants. Most of the antioxidants can help you fight cancer in order to maintain a healthy body. Watermelons, in some localities, are not seasonal and can be purchased year-round. Make sure your watermelons are not spoilt; it should be fresh red.

Pears

Pears are very rich in fiber as well as in Vitamins C. They are reportedly useful in fighting stroke, and eating pears everyday positions your body for better health and longevity. The fiber content of pears afford you the opportunity to speed up your metabolic activities. Pears can be a part of salad or be eaten raw.

Oranges

Oranges have been known for ages as the primary source of Vitamin C that our bodies need. However, it also contains in reasonable amount folate, potassium and fiber. The antioxidants in oranges are very helpful in keeping your skin in good shape.

As you may have discovered in our fruit listing, we provided fruits that are capable of bringing natural growth to your body cells and help you combat several diseases such as cardiac arrest, overweight, diabetes and poor vision.

You may decide to have one or two fruits per day, spread over three squared meals. Do not overeat these fruits in the hope of filling up your body with a lot of nutrients. Just maintain a balanced-diet approach until you can have all of them within a week or more, depending on their availability and your appetite for fruits.

The vegetable listings start from here; we are sure you are familiar with all of them. We refrain from including obscure vegetables in our listing, which readers might have a hard time finding. So, delve right into the list and enjoy yourself reading it!

Garlic

Garlic has enviable medicinal benefits, some of which include but are not restricted to the possession of antioxidants, which help our bodies fight heart diseases and Alzheimer's. Garlic is particularly considered as a memory-boosting veggie! So, apart from its horrid smell, garlic also supplies our bodies with useful nutrients.

Canned Pumpkin

Pumpkins have been known for ages as a real source of antioxidants to human body, and they contain fibers, too, which are very useful in day-to-day metabolic activities. Make sure your canned pumpkin does not contain sodium, which some food companies use as a preservative. Sodium is dangerous to human health.

Canned Tomatoes (Diced)

You will get a good amount of antioxidant lycopene when you consume canned tomatoes. If you are thinking of making fast soup or stew, go for canned tomatoes, but make sure no sodium has been added into the tomatoes as a preservative. Fresh tomatoes are also good; the nutrients are expected to still be in their natural states. You can use canned tomatoes to cook soups, prepare salad and serve as an appetizer!

Onions

You can use onions in a number of ways: as a condiment in vegan dish or soup. Apart from the sharp sensation it invokes on your tongue, onions are also good sources of antioxidants that prevents heart diseases from affecting you. Use your onions as a part of salad or you even choose to chew it. Do not spit out the whorls of the onions, chew everything and swallow it. It is good for your health!

Sweet Potatoes

In addition to its fiber content, sweet potatoes are delicious and very nutritious. They provide Vitamin A to the body and contain beta-carotene, which may hinder the growth of cancerous cells on our skin and protect it from excessive sunlight (tanning). You can decide to make some mashed potatoes or even cooked them as a meal. You may have to combine other vegetables described in this e-book so as to have a great meal.

Winter Squash (Acorn, butternut, etc)

If you are looking for a veggie that can supply your body with freshness, fiber, vitamins and potassium at the same time, go for the winter squash. The primary function of potassium is to help you stay healthy and active by lowering your blood pressure. Imagine how agile you can be when you are not bogged down by a life-threatening high blood pressure!

Kale

If you are looking for a veggie that will supply your body with all the necessary fiber, Vitamins C, A and K, and minerals like calcium, potassium and iron, go for Kale. This veggie is like the superstar of all the nutrient-rich ingredients. Eating kale will help your vision, the growth of your body cells and it will speed up your metabolic processes.

Broccoli

People have been advised from time to time to eat broccoli to fight cancerous cells in their body. Broccoli is also rich in folate and Vitamin C. When you eat broccoli on a regular basis you are protecting your body against a destructive cancer. You can cook your broccoli as a fresh vegetable or you can include it inside a bowl of salad. No matter your choice, it is important to remember that the bottom line is that you are getting as much nutrient as your body required.

Beets

Beets are generally rich in fiber, folate and many vitamins. When you consume beets, you are getting betalains into your body, which is capable of preventing cancer and other body-destroying diseases. Beet can supply magnesium, calcium and iron to your body. Calcium and iron are two elements that are responsible for strengthening some parts of human body, like bones, tendons and muscles.

Spinach

Get Vitamins K and A into your body by eating spinach regularly. This green veggie is also a reservoir of minerals like calcium. Vitamins are good for smooth running of the systems in human bodies. Vitamin A, in particular, is good for maintaining good vision. Spinach has always been included in most salad.

Carrots

This orange veggie is famous for its nutritious components, which include Vitamin A. This vitamin is particularly useful for enjoying a good vision and maintaining smooth skin. Carrots have zero saturated fat and zero cholesterol. It is a typical weight-loss ingredient and it has a considerable amount of fiber.

Edamame

Get it frozen, and you can supply your body with fiber and protein that will help it grow naturally. Edamame is a good source of plant protein! It is a low-calorie vegetable; it also contains Vitamin B complex and calcium. If you want to improve your health, try to eat it at least once a week.

Once again, the good news is that all the healthy fruits and veggies outlined above are cheap to obtain and they are available in all supermarkets all over the world. Get a mix of the fruits and veggies sometimes to increase the amount of minerals and vitamins available to your body at a particular point in time.

We do not encourage abusing foods or fruits: eat as much as you feel is good for your body. It is a wrong notion to think that the larger the quantity of food eaten, the bigger the amount of nutrients that would be assimilated into one's body systems. Food consumption and utilization doesn't work like that; it isn't mathematics that follows a definitive equation formula. Several factors contribute to food utilization in human body: for example, your body systems, your state of health and your willingness to exercise to encourage faster metabolism.

Read This FIRST - 100% FREE BONUS

FOR A LIMITED TIME ONLY – Get Olivia's best-selling book *"The #1 Cookbook: Over 170+ of the Most Popular Recipes Across 7 Different Cuisines!"* absolutely FREE!

Readers have absolutely loved this book because of the wide variety of recipes. It is highly recommended you check these recipes out and see what you can add to your home menu!

Once again, as a big thank-you for downloading this book, I'd like to offer it to you *100% FREE for a LIMITED TIME ONLY!*

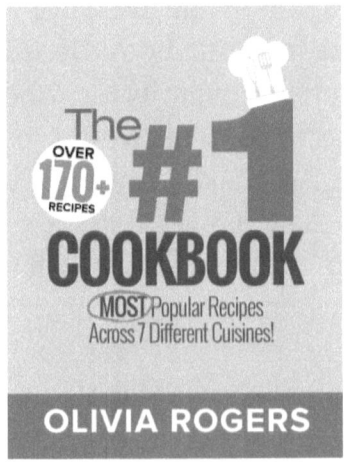

Get your free copy at:

TheMenuAtHome.com/Bonus

Chapter 2: Healthy Proteins

Proteins are integral part of human body, and they are present in our tissues and organs. Proteins are made up of hundreds or thousands of smaller units called amino acids. Amino acids are found in human hair, nails, tendons and other parts. To strengthen our body systems, we definitely need proteins all the time.

Proteins function in different ways in our body: as an antibody for fighting foreign substances that want to attack our health; as an enzyme that facilitates the metabolic processes in our body systems; as a transport/storage facility that helps store up energy for our metabolic activities.

Proteins are obtained from two primary sources: from animals and plants. The healthy proteins included in this e-book are cheap and can be purchased from nearby supermarket. Of course, people don't normally sit down and choose if they were going to buy animal or plant protein. But it is advisable to just mix them up sometimes.

Highlighted below are fourteen healthy proteins you can rely on to transform your health. If you are quite serious about maintaining good health in order to live long, you will surely incorporate these recipes into your daily meals:

Black beans

Black beans are a good source of cancer-killing antioxidants, fiber, and some minerals like calcium, potassium and folic acid. The dry beans are cheaper and they also have their minerals intact. When you boil your black beans, you are inadvertently preserving the antioxidants from being destroyed.

Eggs

Eggs are known as quick suppliers of proteins to human bodies. In other words, when your doctor informed you that your body lacks proteins, go get an egg right away and you will be OK. Eggs seem to possess the same nutrients irrespective of their sources, whether from a fowl or a duck.

Almonds

Almonds contain fiber and monounsaturated fat, the kind of fat that is non-cholesterol in nature. You will probably be advised to eat almonds if you want to fight diabetes and weight-gain. As super-nuts, almonds contribute immensely to the rate of metabolic activity.

Peanuts

Peanuts may be seen as a fatty food but, if eaten moderately, could supply healthy fat to the body. The legumes are good for fighting heart diseases. As a source of plant protein, it is rich in fiber and antioxidants. Do not be tempted to eat plenty of it; it may surprisingly increase the fat in your body.

Garbanzo beans

You can have your Garbanzo beans in a powdery form or as a roast. It contains fiber and it is therefore helpful in speeding up metabolism. It also contains some useful vitamins and minerals such as magnesium and calcium. And it has zero cholesterol but it is rich in dietary fiber.

Lentils

Lentils are used in various meals, as either an ingredient in soup or salad. It is very rich in antioxidants and provides more protein to human body than beef. It tastes good, a quality that makes it popular with vegetarians. Lentils are a low-calorie vegetable and it contains nutrients like calcium, iron and magnesium. The iron and calcium are very useful for strengthening the bones and other structures in human body. Its antioxidant nature helps prevent deadly heart diseases.

Oats

You may have heard that a bowl of oatmeal is a goldmine of health-improving nutrients. You can get fiber, antioxidants and lower-cholesterol fat. Can you imagine how much nutrient you will be able to give your body if you eat oatmeal as your regular breakfast? It also contains minerals like calcium, magnesium, sodium and potassium. Oats also possess some vitamins such as Vitamin B12, B6, D, K, C and A. Vitamin A is good for maintaining a perfect vision while Vitamin C (ascorbic acid) is good for preventing tanning or undue exposure to sunlight.

Pinto beans

You can have your pinto beans for breakfast, lunch and dinner. Pinto beans are very rich in fiber and proteins. The fibers are mainly useful for speeding up metabolic processes. Pinto beans have zero calories and it contains elements like iron, Magnesium, and calcium. The beans also possess some good vitamins such as vitamin B complex, C, D and K, all of which are very helpful in maintaining good health. Do not be afraid to eat these beans in any of your meals, whether during breakfast or other times.

Tofu

Tofu is a soymeal, rich in huge amount of protein but low in fat. Its low-cholesterol characteristic makes it a darling among vegetarians. When consumed moderately, its fiber and antioxidants can reduce cholesterol and the danger of breast cancer.

Pumpkin seeds

If you lack iron, protein and other vitamins in your body, pumpkin seeds can help you replenish them. You can decide to ground it into a powder form or eat it like roasted seeds.

Chicken breasts

A good chicken breast contains lean protein, and you don't have to ever worry about putting on weight when you consumed it. It is important to state that quantity matters: eat a moderate size of the chicken breast and you will just be fine.

Canned salmon

Eat canned salmon to supply your body with the required protein. Canned salmon comes with different flavors, but make sure you select the one with less chemical (food additives) in it.

Canned tuna

The good things about canned tuna is that it is cheap and can provide your body with Omega-3's, which are believed to make people intelligent.

Whey protein

Whey protein can be a good supply of protein to human body when consumed with other foods. For example, you can add it to your bowl of oatmeal or custard.

All the healthy proteins described above are very helpful in speeding up metabolism in humans, and they can be a great anti-aging and anti-cancer agent. Do not be afraid to seek medical assistance from your physician if you do not know which food ingredients will be good for your body or not.

Chapter 3: Healthy Drinks

There are countless drinks around us that are quite unhealthy: they fill up our bodies with excess sugar, fat and cholesterol. In order to remain healthy, it is your singular responsibility to make sure that you only consume drinks that are beneficial to your health, the ones that produce no negative side-effects in your body.

A drink may be regarded as healthy if:

- It doesn't produce too much sugar, fat, cholesterol
- It doesn't contain dangerous additives
- If it is non-alcoholic in nature
- If it facilitates the process of metabolism
- If it is instrumental to weight-loss and mental soberness

The healthy drinks described in this e-book meet all the criteria listed above, and they also contain additional properties that could be regarded to as health-boosting.

Listed below are three main drinks you can drink on a daily basis:

Coffee

Even though it is true that coffee contains caffeine, which is the major reason most people avoid drinking it, but technically, coffee is also a good source of antioxidants which prevent the heart from experiencing cardiac problems. Think of coffee as a fuel for your body when you work out. Home-brewed coffee is more reliable than the one bought from the vending machine or coffee shop. You may not be able to ascertain which ingredients were used in brewing the coffee bought from the coffee shop. Desist from consuming a lot of coffee per day: having a large quantity of caffeine in your blood stream is absolutely bad for your health.

Tea

Tea is reputable for supplying human body with the much-needed antioxidants. Researchers believe that the greener a tea, the more the amount of antioxidants it could release into human body. As long as you didn't put a lot of sugar into your tea, you can enjoy its natural flavor and smell. Drinking green tea, for example, has been noted to improve drinker's immune system and help in maintaining weight. This weight-loss property of green tea is why many people are turning to it as a vital drink to rejuvenate their body system.

Water

We have all seen water as a free substance, which is true to a certain extent. Water is very important for our consumption because human body consists of seventy percent (70%) of water. Water functions as a hydrating liquid that keeps the balance of the metabolites inside the blood stream. Water also helps in flushing out toxic substances from our bodies. If you want to lose weight, drinking some cups of water everyday can position you for a smooth weight-loss process.

Whatever you chose to drink, always remember that you must pay serious attention to the quantity as well as the regularity of consumption. Too much of everything is bad: make sure you consume only the quantity you needed.

Chapter 4: Healthy Whole Grains

Whole grains are notable examples of carbohydrates, and they contain high percentage of dietary fibers per gram. They are also rich in Vitamin B complex (thiamin, riboflavin, niacin and folate). They are noticeable reservoir of life-enriching minerals such as iron, magnesium and selenium.

The primary benefits of whole grains include reducing the chance of contracting a heart disease and facilitating metabolic activities.

If your meal lack whole grains like rice, corns and the others, you better run to the nearest supermarket and grab them. They are very useful for maintaining good health, as you will discover shortly.

In this e-book, we list three essential whole-grain foods for your consumption:

Whole-grain pasta

This white, whole-grain pasta is full of some essential substances like proteins, antioxidants and fiber. When you eat, you aren't only building the cells in your body in a healthy way, but also keeping yourself from having a heart disease.

Brown rice

Brown rice is usually preferred to the white one because it contains a sizeable amount of fiber that is necessary for reducing the risk of diabetes. Most restaurants go for brown rice because of this unique characteristic.

Popcorn

Popcorns are a good source of dietary fiber, and it is always advisable that you to go for the low-calorie ones. Do not mess up your popcorn with too much sugar and other unhealthy additives that some people often add to it.

Chapter 5: Healthy Dairy

While it is a good idea to consume some diary from time to time, the right way to do it is by going for low-fat ones. From milk to yoghurt to cheese, dairy products have been noticed as the main sources of vitamins such as B1, B2, B6, B12, A, E and D and important nutrients like proteins, calcium, folate and magnesium.

Like every other type of food that we consume, here are some significant reasons why people should consume dairy products regularly:

- To replenish our body systems with protein and calcium

- To obtain vitamin D, which is responsible for lowering the risk of cancer

- Calcium from dairy foods are useful for increasing bone density

- Consuming low-fat dairy products prevents high blood pressure from occurring

- Metabolic syndrome, which causes enlarged waists in people, can only affect people who do not eat dairy products

- Dairy products are useful for weight-loss plans

Highlighted below are three important dairy products you can find in any supermarket near you:

Yoghurt

Low-calorie yoghurt is the best choice if you want to maximize the amount of protein and calcium you can derive from it. This type of yoghurt is even helpful in losing weight. Make it your habit to eat it once a day, most especially as part of your breakfast menu.

Low-fat milk

Drink low-fat milk whenever you need to add more calcium and protein to your body system. You can keep your teeth and bone strong by using the calcium supplied by this milk.

Cottage cheese

Cottage cheese is rich in proteins and calcium. It is advisable you go for the low-fat or fat-free one. Cheese often tastes good and you can apply it to different types of meals you have in a day.

Final Words

I would like to thank you for downloading my book and I hope I have been able to help you and educate you about something new.

If you have enjoyed this book and would like to share your positive thoughts, could you please take 30 seconds of your time to go back and give me a review on my Amazon book page!

I greatly appreciate seeing these reviews because it helps me share my hard work!

Again, thank you and I wish you all the best with your cooking journey!

Last Chance to Get YOUR Bonus!

FOR A LIMITED TIME ONLY – Get Olivia's best-selling book *"The #1 Cookbook: Over 170+ of the Most Popular Recipes Across 7 Different Cuisines!"* absolutely FREE!

Readers have absolutely loved this book because of the wide variety of recipes. It is highly recommended you check these recipes out and see what you can add to your home menu!

Once again, as a big thank-you for downloading this book, I'd like to offer it to you *100% FREE for a LIMITED TIME ONLY!*

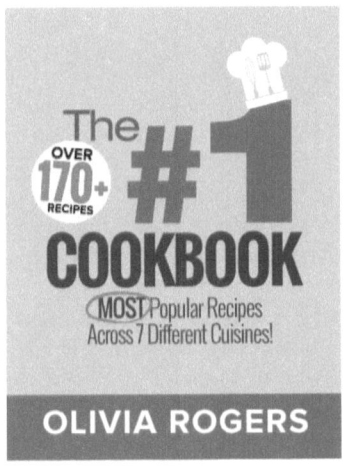

Get your free copy at:

TheMenuAtHome.com/Bonus

Disclaimer

This book and related site provides recipe and food advice in an informative and educational manner only, with information that is general in nature and that is not specific to you, the reader. The contents of this book and related site are intended to assist you and other readers in your personal efforts. Consult your physician or nutritionist regarding the applicability of any information provided in our information to you.

Nothing in this book should be construed as personal advice or diagnosis, and must not be used in this manner. The information provided about conditions is general in nature. This information does not cover all possible uses, actions, precautions, side-effects, or interactions of medicines, or medical procedures. The information in this site should not be considered as complete and does not cover all diseases, ailments, physical conditions, or their treatment.

No Warranties: The authors and publishers don't guarantee or warrant the quality, accuracy, completeness, timeliness, appropriateness or suitability of the information in this book, or of any product or services referenced by this site.

The information in this site is provided on an "as is" basis and the authors and publishers make no representations or warranties of any kind with respect to this information. This site may contain inaccuracies, typographical errors, or other errors.

Liability Disclaimer: The publishers, authors, and other parties involved in the creation, production, provision of information, or delivery of this site specifically disclaim any responsibility, and shall not be held liable for any damages, claims, injuries, losses, liabilities, costs, or obligations including any direct, indirect, special, incidental, or consequences damages (collectively known as "Damages") whatsoever and howsoever caused, arising out of, or in connection with the use or misuse of the site and the information contained within it, whether such Damages arise in contract, tort, negligence, equity, statute law, or by way of other legal theory.

www.ingramcontent.com/pod-product-compliance
Lightning Source LLC
Chambersburg PA
CBHW021135080526
44587CB00012B/1298